Unraveling the hidden world of infections

Emerging threats in Parasitic infection

By

Shirley L. Brooks

Table of content

Introduction

Parasite contamination is a kind of disease brought about by parasites, which are organic entities that live on or inside another life form (the host) and infer their supplements and food from the host. Parasites can be single-celled microorganisms, like protozoa, or multicellular organic entities, like helminths (worms) and arthropods. These parasites can cause a great many illnesses and medical problems in their hosts.

Normal instances of parasitic contamination include the following:

1. Malaria: Brought about by the Plasmodium parasite and communicated by contaminated mosquitoes, intestinal sickness is a hazardous infection that influences a large number of individuals around the world.

2. Giardiasis: This is a digestive disease brought about by the Giardia lamblia parasite, prompting gastrointestinal side effects like loose bowels and stomach torment.

3. Hookworm Disease: Hookworms are parasitic worms that can contaminate the digestive tracts and cause iron deficiency and ailing health.

4. Scabies: This skin invasion is brought about by the Sarcoptes scabiei vermin and prompts extreme tingling and skin rash.

5. Lice Invasion: Head lice and body lice are ectoparasites that swarm the hair and apparel, prompting tingling and uneasiness.

6. Tapeworm Contamination: Taenia and different tapeworms can taint the digestive organs and cause side effects like stomach agony and weight reduction.

Parasitic diseases can be procured through different routes, including ingestion of tainted food or water, contact with contaminated soil, bug nibbles, and close contact with tainted people or creatures.

The avoidance and treatment of parasitic contamination change contingent upon the particular parasite included. Control measures might incorporate drugs, cleanliness practices, and vector control. Understanding and tending to parasitic diseases are fundamental for safeguarding general wellbeing and preventing related medical issues.

The significance of arising parasitic diseases lies in their capability to essentially affect general wellbeing, worldwide economies, and biological systems. Understanding and tending to these arising dangers is essential in light of multiple factors:

1. General Wellbeing Effect: Arising parasitic contaminations can cause far-reaching illness flare-ups, prompting expanded grimness and mortality. These illnesses can overpower medical care frameworks and have extreme ramifications for impacted people and networks.

2. Globalization and Travel: In our interconnected world, irresistible sicknesses, including parasitic diseases, can immediately spread across borders through global travel and exchange. This makes arising diseases a worldwide worry, as they can influence individuals in different regions of the planet.

3. Environmental Change: Changes in the environment, for example, can impact the appropriation and conduct of parasites and their vectors. Changes in temperature and precipitation can create conditions that favor the endurance and transmission of parasites, prompting the rise of illnesses in districts where they were previously absent.

4. Drug Obstruction: Parasites have created protection from ordinarily utilized antiparasitic drugs. The rise of medication-safe strains can confuse treatment and control endeavors, making it critical to foster new drugs and techniques.

5. Dismissed Sicknesses: Arising dangers can incorporate dismissed tropical illnesses (NTDs), which lopsidedly influence devastated locales. The resurgence or expanded rate of NTDs is a central issue for worldwide wellbeing value and the social turn of events.

6. Zoonotic Potential: Many arising parasitic diseases are zoonotic, meaning they can be transmitted among creatures and people. This features the significance of a One Wellbeing approach that thinks about the interconnectedness of human, creature, and natural wellbeing.

7. Challenges in Conclusion and Treatment: Rising contaminations frequently present symptomatic and treatment challenges. Medical care frameworks may not be ready to recognize and deal with these illnesses, requiring exploration and foundation enhancements.

8. Examination and Reconnaissance: Arising parasitic diseases require continuous exploration to figure out their elements and foster compelling control techniques. Reconnaissance is critical to recognizing and screening for these contaminations as soon as possible.

9. Monetary Effect: Arising parasitic contaminations can upset agrarian efficiency and impede the monetary turn of events, especially in districts vigorously dependent on farming. This can prompt expanded destitution and social flimsiness.

10. Biodiversity and Biological System Wellbeing: Parasitic contaminations can influence untamed life and environmental wellbeing. Understanding and alleviating arising parasitic contaminations are fundamental for protecting biodiversity and biological system administrations.

In outline, arising parasitic contaminations are critical because of their capability to disturb general wellbeing, economies, and environments. Watchfulness, research, observation, worldwide joint effort, and the advancement of successful anticipation and control systems are fundamental to addressing these developing dangers to human and creature wellbeing.

Chapter 1: The Elements of Arising Parasites

The elements of arising parasites are perplexing and multi-layered, formed by a scope of variables that impact their commonness, transmission, and effect on human and creature populations. Understanding these elements is pivotal for the powerful administration and control of arising parasitic contaminations. Here are a few critical elements of arising parasites:

1. Resurgence and New Geographic Areas: Arising parasites might return in regions where they were recently controlled or totally missing. This resurgence can be due to different elements, including changes in the environment, human movement, and the unwinding of control measures.

2. Vector Elements: Numerous parasitic diseases are communicated by vectors, like mosquitoes, ticks, or insects. Changes in vector behavior and circulation can impact the spread of parasites. For instance, changes in temperature and precipitation can influence the reach and movement of sickness vectors.

3. Zoonotic Potential: Arising parasites frequently have zoonotic potential, meaning they can be communicated among creatures and people. This powerful feature highlights the significance of a One Wellbeing approach that thinks about the interconnectedness of human, creature, and ecological wellbeing.

4. Hereditary Variety and Medication Opposition: Parasites can quickly advance and adjust to evolving conditions. Hereditary variety inside parasite populations can prompt the development of medication-safe strains, making treatment and control really testing.

5. Natural Changes: Changes in the climate, like deforestation, urbanization, and horticultural practices, can create natural

surroundings that favor the endurance and transmission of parasites. Ecological changes can likewise disturb the normal harmony between hosts, parasites, and vectors.

6. Human Way of Behaving and Financial Variables: Human activities, like travel, exchange, and urbanization, assume a huge part in the spread of arising parasites. Financial variables, including neediness and admittance to medical care, can impact the risk of parasitic diseases.

7. Environmental Change: Environmental change can straightforwardly affect the appropriation of parasites and their vectors. Increasing temperatures and adjusted precipitation examples can extend the topographical scope of parasitic contamination and influence the planning of infection transmission.

8. Globalization and Travel: Expanded worldwide travel and exchange work with the acquaintance of parasites in new areas. Individuals, creatures, and merchandise can act as accidental transporters of parasites, prompting the acquaintance of sicknesses with already unaffected regions.

9. Vector Control and Infection The executives: Control measures, for example, vector control and medication organization, can impact the elements of arising parasites. Conflicting or inadequate control endeavors can contribute to the reappearance of illnesses.

10. Examination and Reconnaissance: Continuous examination and observation are vital for screening and grasping the elements of arising parasites. This data is significant for creating compelling counteraction and control techniques.

In synopsis, the elements of the arising parasites are impacted by a perplexing transaction of natural, organic, ecological, and sociodemographic factors. A complete and multidisciplinary approach is important to address and deal with these unique difficulties for general wellbeing and biological system prosperity.

The Elements of Arising Parasites

The elements of arising parasites are perplexing and multi-layered, formed by a scope of variables that impact their commonness, transmission, and effect on human and creature populations. Understanding these elements is pivotal for the powerful administration and control of arising parasitic contaminations. Here are a few critical elements of arising parasites:

1. Resurgence and New Geographic Areas: Arising parasites might return in regions where they were recently controlled or totally missing. This resurgence can be due to different elements, including changes in the environment, human movement, and the unwinding of control measures.

2. Vector Elements: Numerous parasitic diseases are communicated by vectors, like mosquitoes, ticks, or insects. Changes in vector behavior and circulation can impact the spread of parasites. For instance, changes in temperature and precipitation can influence the reach and movement of sickness vectors.

3. Zoonotic Potential: Arising parasites frequently have zoonotic potential, meaning they can be communicated among creatures and people. This powerful feature highlights the significance of a One Wellbeing approach that thinks about the interconnectedness of human, creature, and ecological wellbeing.

4. Hereditary Variety and Medication Opposition: Parasites can quickly advance and adjust to evolving conditions. Hereditary variety inside parasite populations can prompt the development

of medication-safe strains, making treatment and control really testing.

5. Natural Changes: Changes in the climate, like deforestation, urbanization, and horticultural practices, can create natural surroundings that favor the endurance and transmission of parasites. Ecological changes can likewise disturb the normal harmony between hosts, parasites, and vectors.

6. Human Way of Behaving and Financial Variables: Human activities, like travel, exchange, and urbanization, assume a huge part in the spread of arising parasites. Financial variables, including neediness and admittance to medical care, can impact the risk of parasitic diseases.

7. Environmental Change: Environmental change can straightforwardly affect the appropriation of parasites and their vectors. Increasing temperatures and adjusted precipitation examples can extend the topographical scope of parasitic contamination and influence the planning of infection transmission.

8. Globalization and Travel: Expanded worldwide travel and exchange work with the acquaintance of parasites in new areas. Individuals, creatures, and merchandise can act as accidental transporters of parasites, prompting the acquaintance of sicknesses with already unaffected regions.

9. Vector Control and Infection The executives: Control measures, for example, vector control and medication organization, can impact the elements of arising parasites. Conflicting or inadequate control endeavors can contribute to the reappearance of illnesses.

10. Examination and Reconnaissance: Continuous examination and observation are vital for screening and grasping the elements of arising parasites. This data is significant for creating compelling counteraction and control techniques.

In synopsis, the elements of the arising parasites are impacted by a perplexing transaction of natural, organic, ecological, and sociodemographic factors. A complete and multidisciplinary approach is important to address and deal with these unique difficulties for general wellbeing and biological system prosperity.

Factors adding to their development

The development of parasitic contamination is impacted by various complex elements. While the particular causes can differ contingent upon the parasite and the locale, coming up next are a few normal elements contributing to the development of parasitic diseases:

1. Environmental Change: Modifications in temperature, precipitation examples, and stickiness can influence the conveyance of parasites and their vectors. Environmental change can create conditions that favor the endurance and transmission of parasites in new geographic districts.

2. Natural Changes: Changes in land use, like deforestation, urbanization, and farming practices, can adjust the climate and create natural surroundings that help the spread of parasites. For instance, the making of fake water supplies can give favorable places to parasites like mosquitoes.

3. Vector Elements: Parasitic contaminations frequently rely upon vectors, like mosquitoes, ticks, and flies, to communicate the parasites to humans. Changes in the dispersion and conduct of these vectors, affected by factors like the environment, can affect the spread of parasitic illnesses.

4. Globalization and Travel: Expanded global travel, exchange, and development of individuals and products can acquaint parasites with new regions. Parasites can be conveyed by contaminated people, creatures, or imported items.

5. Zoonotic Potential: Many emerging parasites are zoonotic, meaning they can taint both creatures and people. The overflow of parasites from untamed life or homegrown creatures to people can prompt the development of new infections.

6. Drug Obstruction: The improvement of medication resistance in parasites is a critical concern. Abuse or abuse of antiparasitic medications can prompt the determination of safe strains, making treatment less successful.

7. Financial Elements: Neediness, absence of access to clean water and sterilization, and restricted medical services assets can create conditions that favor the development and ingenuity of parasitic diseases.

8. Human Way of Behaving: Travel, movement, and changes in the human way of behaving can expand openness to parasitic diseases. For instance, travel to endemic districts without legitimate safety measures can bring about the acquaintance of parasites with new regions.

9. Absence of Reconnaissance and Control: Deficient reconnaissance and control measures can add to the resurgence of parasitic diseases. This might happen because of an absence of assets, foundation, or mindfulness.

10. Anti-microbial Use in Horticulture: The utilization of anti-toxins in agribusiness can influence the stomach microbiota of domesticated animals and effect the presence and transmission of parasitic contamination.

11. Vector Control Practices: Conflicting or ineffectual vector control measures can permit vectors to multiply, prompting expanded transmission of parasitic sicknesses.

12. Struggle and Uprooting: Furnished clashes and populace dislodging can upset medical care frameworks and create conditions that favor the spread of parasitic diseases.

13. Natural Awkwardness: Changes in the regular harmony between hosts, parasites, and vectors can prompt the development of parasitic contamination in new regions.

Understanding these contributing variables and their associations is vital for anticipating, forestalling, and dealing with the rise of parasitic diseases and for creating successful control and moderation systems.

Chapter 2: Intestinal Sickness and Resurgence

Jungle fever resurgence alludes to the return or expansion in the rate of jungle fever in districts where it was beforehand taken care of, or a resurgence of cases in regions with a past decrease in intestinal sickness transmission. This peculiarity has been a critical worry in the field of general wellbeing because of its effect on impacted populations and the difficulties it presents in the battle against this lethal sickness. A few variables contribute to the jungle fever resurgence:

1. Drug Obstruction: The improvement of medication-safe jungle fever parasites, for example, Plasmodium falciparum, has been a main consideration in the intestinal sickness resurgence. Protection from antimalarial drugs, like chloroquine and sulfadoxine-pyrimethamine, has made these medications less powerful in treating the illness.

1. Vector Obstruction: Anopheles mosquitoes, the essential vectors of jungle fever, have created protection from insect poisons utilized in vector control programs. This opposition lessens the viability of techniques like indoor lingering showering and insect spray-treated bed nets.

2. Feeble Wellbeing Frameworks: In districts with frail medical services foundation, observation, and therapy limits, the capacity to distinguish and answer jungle fever cases is restricted. This can prompt unrestrained transmission and a resurgence of the sickness.

3. Environmental Change: Changes in temperature and precipitation can influence the rearing and endurance of mosquitoes, adjusting the circulation and transmission of jungle fever. Hotter and wetter circumstances can expand the geographic scope of intestinal sickness, adding to the resurgence.

4. Human Relocation: Population developments, whether because of contention, monetary elements, or natural changes, can acquaint jungle fever with new regions or once again introduce it to previously intestinal sickness-free districts. Travelers from endemic regions might carry the sickness with them.

5. Protection from Control Measures: Intestinal sickness parasites and vectors can adjust to control estimates after some time. This can reflect changes in mosquito conduct, making them more dynamic during times when control measures are less viable.

6. Lack of concern and diminished subsidizing: At the point when jungle fever is effectively controlled, there might be a decrease in financing and consideration regarding the sickness, prompting an unwinding of control endeavors. This lack of concern can make us ready for a resurgence.

7. Monetary Effect: The jungle fever resurgence can thwart monetary advancement by expanding medical care costs, lessening efficiency, and causing financial shakiness in impacted locales.

Endeavors to battle the jungle fever resurgence incorporate the turn of events and arrangement of new antimalarial drugs, investigation into insect poison opposition, fortifying medical care frameworks, and advancing the supportable utilization of vector control strategies. The jungle fever resurgence highlights the significance of supported venture, exploration, and watchfulness in the battle against this preventable and treatable sickness.

Chapter 3: Environmental Change and Parasites

Environmental change altogether affects the conveyance, conduct, and pervasiveness of parasites, remembering those that cause different irresistible sicknesses for people, creatures, and plants. Parasitic creatures are exceptionally delicate to natural circumstances, and, surprisingly, slight adjustments in temperature, dampness, and precipitation can create conditions that are better for their endurance and transmission. Here are the critical ways in which environmental change impacts parasites:

1. Change in Geographic Conveyance: As temperatures climb and nearby environments change, the geographic scope of numerous parasites and their vectors (e.g., mosquitoes, ticks) can grow. Parasites that were recently bound to explicit locales may now track down appropriate circumstances in new regions, prompting the acquaintance of sicknesses with beforehand unaffected districts.

2. Changed Transmission Elements: Environmental change can influence the irregularity and power of parasitic diseases. Changes in temperature and mugginess can impact the turn of events and endurance of parasites inside their vectors and hosts, influencing transmission designs.

3. Vector-Borne Illnesses: Numerous parasitic illnesses, like intestinal sickness and dengue fever, are transmitted by vectors like mosquitoes. Climbing temperatures can accelerate the improvement of parasites inside these vectors, prompting expanded transmission rates.

4. Vector Conduct: Environmental change can impact the way in which illness vectors behave. For example, adjusted temperature and mugginess might urge mosquitoes to chomp all the more every now and again or at various times, which can influence the risk of vector-borne infections.

5. Infection Resurgence: As parasites extend their reach into new regions, districts that were already liberated from specific parasitic illnesses might encounter an infection resurgence. This can surprise medical service frameworks and require new control procedures.

6. Impacts on Untamed Life: Environmental change can influence untamed life populations and their parasites. For example, hotter temperatures can prompt the multiplication of specific parasites in sea-going environments, affecting fish and land and water proficient populations.

7. Collaborations with Hosts: Changed natural circumstances can influence the resistant reaction and helplessness of hosts to parasitic contamination. Environmental change can impact parasite collaborations in ways that influence illness elements.

8. Plant Parasites: Crop sicknesses brought about by plant parasites can likewise be affected by environmental change. Hotter temperatures and changes in precipitation can influence the predominance and seriousness of these contaminations, affecting food security.

9. Environment Effect: Changes in parasitic diseases can influence environmental wellbeing and biodiversity. Parasites assume fundamental parts in biological system elements, and changes in parasite-have connections can have flowing consequences for environments.

10. Influence on Animals: Parasitic diseases in domesticated animals can lessen rural efficiency. Environmental change might modify the appropriation and weight of these contaminations, influencing the cultivation of domesticated animals.

Endeavors to relieve the effect of environmental change on parasites and irresistible illnesses incorporate checking and reconnaissance programs, variation methodologies for medical services frameworks, examination into the changing elements of sicknesses, and measures to control infection vectors. Tending to environmental change and its consequences for parasitic contamination is pivotal for the wellbeing and prosperity of people, creatures, and biological systems.

The role of environmental change in the spread of parasitic diseases

Environmental change assumes a critical role in the spread of parasitic contamination, influencing the circulation, transmission, and prevalence of different parasitic illnesses. The connection between environmental change and parasitic diseases is intricate and diverse. Here are key ways in which environmental change impacts the spread of parasitic diseases:

1. Adjusted Geographic Appropriation: Climbing temperatures and changing precipitation examples can create new environments for parasites and their vectors. Parasites that were once restricted to explicit areas might grow their geographic reach as conditions become more appropriate for their endurance and multiplication. This can acquaint illnesses with new regions and increase the risk of disease.

2. Vector-Borne Illnesses: Numerous parasitic contaminations are transmitted by vectors like mosquitoes, ticks, and flies. Environmental change can influence the dispersion and conduct of these vectors. Hotter temperatures can speed up the improvement of parasites inside vectors, increase the life expectancy of vectors, and lead to more regular blood-taking, all of which contribute to higher transmission rates.

3. Change in Irregularity: Changes in the environment can modify the irregularity of parasitic illnesses. Hotter winters and expanded transmission seasons can bring about longer periods of likely openness to irresistible specialists, prompting expanded infection transmission.

4. Vector Conveyance: Changes in temperature and stickiness can affect the circulation of illness vectors. Vectors might move to higher elevations or scopes, growing the regions where they can communicate sickness.

5. Vector Conduct: Environmental change can impact the way in which illness vectors behave. For instance, hotter temperatures might urge vectors to take care of themselves all the more every now and again, chomp at various times, or change their host inclinations. These social changes can influence the risk of transmission.

6. Waterborne Parasites: Parasitic contaminations sent through water, for example, those brought about by protozoa like Giardia and Cryptosporidium, can be impacted by changes in water quality and accessibility driven by environmental change.

7. Have Parasite Associations: Environmental change can impact parasite communications, influencing the defenselessness and insusceptible reactions of host species. This can affect elements of illness, especially in natural life populations.

8. Infection Resurgence: Parasitic illnesses might resurge in districts where they were recently controlled because of changing natural circumstances. This resurgence can surprise medical service frameworks and require new control methodologies.

9. Ignored Tropical Illnesses: Environmental change can fuel the weight of ignored tropical sicknesses (NTDs) in endemic districts, where neediness and restricted admittance to medical care assets as of now add to illness transmission.

10. Plant Parasites: Parasitic contamination in plants and yields can be impacted by environmental change. Changes in temperature and precipitation can influence the pervasiveness and seriousness of harvest illnesses, affecting food security.

11. Environment Effect: Environmental change can influence biological system wellbeing and biodiversity. Modifications in parasite-have connections can have flowing consequences for biological systems, affecting natural life populations and environmental elements.

Endeavors to relieve the effect of environmental change on parasitic contaminations incorporate checking and observation programs, variation techniques for medical services frameworks, investigation into the changing elements of infections, and measures to control sickness vectors. Tending to environmental change and its consequences for parasitic contamination is pivotal for the wellbeing and prosperity of people, creatures, and biological systems.

Influence on parasite dispersion and infection designs

Environmental change can significantly affect parasite dispersion and sickness designs, impacting the commonality, geographic reach, and irregularity of different parasitic contaminations. These progressions can have critical ramifications for general wellbeing, environments, and farming. This is the way environmental change influences parasite appropriation and sickness designs:

1. Extended Geographic Reach: Climbing temperatures can create better circumstances for parasites and their vectors in locales where they were already extraordinary or missing. This development of appropriate natural surroundings can bring about the acquaintance of parasitic infections with new regions.

2. Change in Elevation and Scope: Changes in temperature and dampness can prompt the development of parasites at higher elevations and scopes. This shift can expose previously uninfected populations to parasitic diseases.

3. Vector-Borne Illnesses: Numerous parasites, like those causing intestinal sickness, dengue fever, and Lyme illness, are communicated by vectors like mosquitoes and ticks. Environmental change can modify the conveyance and conduct of these vectors, expanding the risk of transmission and broadening the transmission season.

4. Changes in Irregularity: Hotter winters and stretched-out transmission seasons can prompt a more drawn-out period during which individuals, creatures, and untamed life are in danger of contamination. This can influence sickness examples and lead to expanded instances of specific parasitic contamination.

5. Changed Transmission Elements: Parasite transmission can be affected by temperature-subordinate variables, including the advancement of parasites inside vectors. As temperatures climb, parasites might breed all the more rapidly, prompting higher disease rates in vectors and hosts.

6. Waterborne Parasites: Environmental change can influence water quality and the accessibility of freshwater assets. Parasitic diseases communicated through sullied water, for example, those brought about by protozoa like Giardia and Cryptosporidium, can turn out to be more prevalent under changing hydrological conditions.

7. Change in Natural Life Sickness Elements: Environmental change can influence the strength of untamed life populations by modifying the dispersion and pervasiveness of parasitic infections among creatures. These progressions can have flowing consequences for biological systems and untamed life preservation endeavors.

8. Ignored Tropical Illnesses: Districts previously troubled by ignored tropical infections (NTDs) may encounter expanded transmission because of the evolving environment. Neediness and restricted access to medical services assets here can worsen the effect of NTDs.

9. Crop Sicknesses: Parasitic diseases in plants and harvests can be impacted by temperature and precipitation changes. This can prompt adjusted infection examples and affect food security.

10. Financial Results: Changes in parasite dissemination and sickness examples can have monetary ramifications, for example, diminished rural efficiency, expanded medical service costs, and the possible disturbance of exchange and the travel industry.

Endeavors to address the effect of environmental change on parasite circulation and sickness designs incorporate reconnaissance and checking programs, advancement of versatile methodologies for medical services frameworks, examination into the changing elements of illnesses, and measures to control infection vectors. Understanding and getting ready for these progressions is essential to moderate the impacts of environmental change on general wellbeing, biological systems, and agribusiness.

Chapter 4: Ignored Tropical Infections

Ignored Tropical Sicknesses (NTDs) address a gathering of different irresistible infections that principally burden the world's most devastated and minimized populations. These illnesses, frequently disregarded by medical care frameworks and worldwide wellbeing drives, flourish in regions with restricted access to clean water, sterilization, and medical services assets. Here is an outline of NTDs:

1. Pervasiveness and Geographic Dispersion:

• NTDs are pervasive in tropical and subtropical locales of the world, particularly in low- and middle-income nations.

• More than a billion people are impacted by NTDs, with the majority living in sub-Saharan Africa, Asia, and Latin America.

2. Various Gatherings of Sicknesses:

• NTDs envelop a great many illnesses, including helminth contaminations (for example, soil-communicated helminthiasis and schistosomiasis), protozoal diseases (like African resting disorder and Chagas sickness), bacterial contaminations (uncleanliness and Buruli ulcer), and viral diseases (dengue fever).

3. Method of Transmission:

• NTDs are communicated through different means, including defiled water and soil, vector-borne transmission (through bugs), and direct contact with contaminated people or creatures.

4. Constant and Incapacitating

• NTDs can cause constant and crippling side effects, including serious agony, distortion, visual deficiency, mental debilitation, and actual incapacities.

• They add to a pattern of destitution by diminishing efficiency and ruining the monetary turn of events.

5. Influence on General Wellbeing:

• NTDs can significantly affect general wellbeing. They frequently lead to dreariness, long-term incapacity, and demise, especially when left untreated.

• These infections lopsidedly influence kids, ladies, and weak populaces.

6. Shame and Segregation:

• Numerous NTDs convey social disgrace and segregation, frequently disengaging impacted people from their networks and restricting their access to school and work.

7. Covering contaminations:

• Co-diseases are normal among people in endemic districts, intensifying the wellbeing of NTDs.

• The exchange among NTDs and other irresistible illnesses, similar to HIV and tuberculosis, presents complex wellbeing challenges.

8. Anticipation and Control:

• Deterrent measures for NTDs incorporate mass medication organization, further developed sterilization and cleanliness, vector control, and wellbeing instruction.

• Multisectoral approaches, including the coordination of NTD control with other wellbeing and improvement programs, are fundamental.

9. Worldwide Drives:

• Associations like the World Wellbeing Association (WHO) and non-legislative associations are effectively engaged in endeavors to control and take out NTDs.

• The London Statement on NTDs and the 2030 NTD Guide provide vital structures for tending to these infections.

10. Progress and Difficulties:

• Critical headway has been made in diminishing the pervasiveness of some NTDs, yet challenges remain, including financing holes, admittance to medical care in far-off regions, and guaranteeing that NTD programs are practical.
• Tending to NTDs is critical for achieving worldwide wellbeing value and decreasing destitution. By focusing on exploration, financing, and composed endeavors, the worldwide local area intends to control, kill, or annihilate NTDs and further develop the prosperity of those impacted by these overwhelming infections.

Arising Disregarded Tropical Sicknesses (NTDs) and Difficulties in Charge

Arising NTDs are illnesses that have, as of late, expanded in frequency or extended their geographic reach, presenting new difficulties to general wellbeing. These illnesses frequently influence underestimated and weak populations in tropical and subtropical locales. Here are some arising NTDs and the difficulties in their control:

1. Zika Infection Disease:

• Challenge: Zika infection has arisen as a huge danger because of its relationship with birth surrenders (microcephaly) in babies. Controlling Zika requires hearty mosquito control measures and safe regenerative wellbeing practices to decrease the risk of transmission.

2. Lymphatic filariasis (LF):

• Challenge: LF is a laid-out NTD, yet its disposal has been tested by causing drug obstruction in certain areas. Progressing research is expected to foster elective treatment procedures.

3. Leishmaniasis:

• Challenge: Cutaneous and instinctive leishmaniasis have extended their geographic ranges and are progressively influencing non-endemic districts. Environmental change and human movement add to this spread.

4. Mycetoma:

• Challenge: Mycetoma is a constant skin and delicate tissue contamination with restricted treatment choices. Further developed diagnostics and reasonable, successful medicines are required.

5. Snakebite envenoming:

• Challenge: Snakebite envenoming has earned respect as a NTD because of its dangerous effect on rustic networks. Challenges include further developing admittance to antibody and medical care administrations for far-off regions.

6. Arising Helminth Contaminations:

• Challenge: Helminthic parasites like schistosomes and soil-sent helminths keep on presenting difficulties in charge, especially with the advancement of medication resistance in certain areas.

7. Wellbeing Framework Fortifying:

• Challenge: Many arising NTDs require reinforced medical services frameworks, including expanded admittance to medical services offices and prepared staff. This can be tried in asset-obligated settings.

8. Environmental Change and Vector Control:

• Challenge: Environmental change can affect the circulation and conduct of sickness vectors. Fighting arising NTDs requires adjusting vector control measures to evolving conditions.

9. Admittance to Treatment and Anticipation:

• Challenge: Guaranteeing admittance to treatment and counteraction estimates in remote and underestimated networks remains a test. This incorporates giving mass medication organization, safe water, and disinfection.

10. Innovative work:

• Challenge: Examination to comprehend the science and study of disease transmission in arising NTDs is urgent. Growing new demonstrative instruments and viable medicines is much of the time ruined by restricted subsidizing and consideration.

11. Reconnaissance and Revealing:

• Challenge: Solid reconnaissance frameworks are fundamental for following arising NTDs. Further developing detailing and information assortment in low-asset settings is testing yet crucial.

12. Worldwide coordinated effort and subsidizing:

• Challenge: Satisfactory subsidizing and global joint effort are critical for tending to arising NTDs. These infections frequently get less consideration and financing compared with other worldwide medical problems.

Endeavors to control arising NTDs require a multidisciplinary approach, including legislatures, worldwide associations, scientists, and impacted networks. By tending to these difficulties, the worldwide local area can pursue forestalling and controlling arising NTDs and working on the wellbeing and prosperity of those impacted.

Chapter 5: Urbanization and Parasitic Contaminations

Urbanization, the course of populace movement from country to metropolitan region, altogether affects parasitic diseases. While urbanization can prompt better access to medical care, sterilization, and everyday environments, it also achieves different changes that impact the transmission of parasitic contamination. Here are a few critical patterns and their effect on parasitic contamination in metropolitan regions:

1. Expanded Admittance to Medical Care:

• Influence: Urbanization frequently prompts better admittance to medical care offices, which can work on the determination and therapy of parasitic diseases.

• Challenge: Metropolitan medical services frameworks might in any case confront difficulties in tending to the exceptional necessities of metropolitan populaces, including irresistible illnesses that are more pervasive in rustic regions.

2. Further developed sanitation and cleanliness:

• Influence: Metropolitan regions, for the most part, have better sterilization and cleanliness foundations, lessening the risk of waste oral and waterborne parasitic contamination.

• Challenge: While sterilization is improved, there might in any case be pockets of lacking disinfection in metropolitan ghettos, which can prompt limited flare-ups of contaminations like cholera and intestinal parasites.

3. Vector-Borne Contaminations:

• Influence: Urbanization can adjust the natural surroundings of illness vectors, like mosquitoes and rodents. This can influence the transmission of vector-borne parasitic illnesses like intestinal sickness and dengue fever.

• Challenge: Fast urbanization can make favorable places for illness vectors, especially in regions with unfortunate waste administration and standing water, prompting expanded sickness transmission.

4. Relocation and Globalization:

• Influence: Metropolitan regions are center points for relocation and global travel, expanding the risk of presenting parasitic diseases from different districts.

• Challenge: Parasites that were once restricted to explicit geographic locales can spread to metropolitan regions, requiring carefulness regarding analysis, observation, and control.

5. Swarmed day-to-day environments:

• Influence: Metropolitan regions can have thickly populated areas and swarmed everyday environments. This can work with the transmission of a few parasitic diseases, especially those spread through close contact or tainted surfaces.

• Challenge: Congestion can expand the risk of episodes, like scabies or lice pervasions, in metropolitan settings.

6. Food and Waterborne Diseases:

• Influence: Urbanization can expand the accessibility of handled and road food, which might represent a gamble for foodborne parasitic diseases.

• Challenge: Metropolitan populations might have restricted access to safe drinking water, and pollution of water sources can prompt waterborne parasitic diseases.

7. Ignored Tropical Illnesses (NTDs):

• Influence: Some NTDs are more normal in metropolitan ghettos, where unfortunate everyday environments and restricted access to medical care prevail.

• Challenge: Metropolitan NTD control programs should be customized to the unique difficulties of metropolitan regions, including arriving at minimized populations.

8. Environment and Ecological Changes:

• Influence: Urbanization can change neighborhood environments and conditions, which might impact the presence and conduct of sickness vectors and parasites.

• Challenge: These progressions can prompt the rise or reappearance of parasitic diseases, requiring versatile control measures.

Urbanization patterns affect parasitic contamination. While metropolitan regions offer better everyday environments and access to medical care, they likewise present remarkable difficulties for the control and anticipation of parasitic diseases, particularly in regions with a deficient foundation or rapid population development. Successful general wellbeing methodologies should address the particular requirements and dangers related to urbanization to diminish the weight of parasitic diseases in metropolitan settings.

The special difficulties of metropolitan parasitology

Metropolitan parasitology, the investigation of parasitic contaminations in metropolitan settings, presents a few novel difficulties that vary from those experienced in rustic or far-off regions. These moves emerge because of the particular qualities of metropolitan conditions and populations. Here are a portion of the special difficulties of metropolitan parasitology:

1. Different Population and Movement:

• Metropolitan regions frequently have exceptionally assorted populations, including travelers from various areas and nations. This variety can present many parasitic contaminations, making observation and finding more mind-boggling.

2. Overcrowding:

• Packed everyday environments in metropolitan ghettos and casual settlements can help with the quick spread of parasitic diseases that are communicated through close contact, polluted water, or unfortunate sterilization.

3. Restricted Admittance to Clean Water and Sterilization:

• While metropolitan regions by and large have better access to clean water and disinfection than rustic areas, a lack of framework in a few metropolitan areas can in any case prompt waterborne and waste oral parasitic diseases.

4. Vector-Borne Contaminations:

• Urbanization can change the territories of illness vectors, for example, mosquitoes and rodents, possibly expanding the transmission of vector-borne parasitic illnesses like intestinal sickness and dengue fever.

5. Ignored Tropical Illnesses (NTDs):

• Some NTDs are more common in metropolitan ghettos, where restricted access to medical services, sterilization, and cleanliness increases the risk of transmission. NTD control programs should adjust to metropolitan settings.

6. Co-diseases and comorbidities:

• Metropolitan populations might encounter a higher burden of irresistible illnesses, including parasitic contamination. Co-diseases and comorbidities can muddle analysis and treatment.

7. Absence of Mindfulness and Wellbeing in Schooling:

• Quick urbanization can prompt chronic weakness education and attention to parasitic contamination. Individuals in metropolitan regions may not perceive the signs and side effects of parasitic illnesses, prompting deferred conclusions and therapy.

8. Admittance to Medical Care Administrations:

• While metropolitan regions commonly have medical care offices, underestimated populations in metropolitan ghettos may, in any case, confront hindrances to getting to medical services administrations. Disgrace, cost, and distance can restrict medical care usage.

9. Globalization and Travel:

• Metropolitan regions are center points for worldwide travel and movement. This can present parasitic diseases from different locales and pose difficulties regarding conclusion and reconnaissance.

10. Complex Financial Variables:

• Metropolitan parasitology is impacted by a mind-boggling interchange of financial variables, including neediness, imbalance, and business conditions. These elements can increase the risk of parasitic diseases.

11. Natural Changes:

• Urbanization can prompt natural adjustments that impact the presence and conduct of infection vectors and parasites. Environmental change, changes in water bodies, and metropolitan improvements can affect transmission elements.

12. Coordinated Approaches:

• Control and avoidance systems in metropolitan parasitology frequently require coordinated approaches that think about medical services as well as ecological administration, lodging conditions, and the financial turn of events.

Tending to these interesting difficulties of metropolitan parasitology requires custom-made general wellbeing procedures that think about the metropolitan setting, adjust to neighborhood conditions, and draw in networks to further develop admittance to medical care and advance wellbeing mindfulness. It likewise underlines the significance of examination, reconnaissance, and coordinated effort between legislatures, non-administrative associations, and medical services suppliers to control and forestall parasitic contaminations in metropolitan regions successfully.

Chapter 6: Globalization and Travel-Related Diseases

Globalization, as described by expanded worldwide travel, exchange, and interconnectedness, has had a huge impact on the spread of parasites and the illnesses they cause. The development of individuals, creatures, and merchandise across borders has worked with the transmission of parasitic diseases, and this peculiarity presents a few key elements contributing to the spread of parasites:

1. Worldwide travel and the travel industry:

• Expanded travel permits people to convey parasitic contaminations across nations and landmasses. Vacationers and business explorers can become tainted in one locale and communicate the contamination to their nation of origin.

2. Movement and Relocation:

• Movement, whether because of contention, monetary variables, or natural changes, can acquaint parasitic diseases with new regions. Travelers might convey parasites from their home areas to their objective nations.

3. Imported Items and Vector Presentation:

• Contaminated creatures, plants, or items can acquaint infection vectors or parasites with new regions. For instance, the importation of outlandish pets or plants can prompt the presentation of infections conveyed by parasites.

4. Food and Waterborne Diseases:

• Worldwide exchange of food items can bring about the transmission of parasites through polluted food and water. Imported food sources might be wellsprings of parasitic contamination while possibly not being sufficiently observed and controlled.

5. Intrusive species and zoonotic contamination:

• The worldwide development of intrusive species can acquaint diseases with new biological systems. A few parasites are communicated among creatures and people (zoonotic contaminations), and these can be conveyed by untamed life or trained creatures across borders.

6. Drug Opposition and Treatment Difficulties:

• Worldwide drug exchange and the development of individuals can contribute to the spread of medication-safe types of parasites. Treatment challenges emerge when drug-safe parasites are acquainted with new districts.

7. Vector-Borne Illnesses:

• Globalization can adjust the circulation of sickness vectors (e.g., mosquitoes, ticks), which transmit parasitic diseases. Changes in vector conduct and circulation can extend the geographic scope of these illnesses.

8. Environmental Change and Natural Effects:

• Globalization adds to environmental change, which can influence the territories of sickness vectors and the endurance of parasites. As parasites adjust to evolving conditions, they might move to new locales.

9. Ignored Tropical Illnesses (NTDs):

• NTDs, common in low- and middle-income nations, can be spread to different locales by explorers and transients. They are much of the time ignored in worldwide wellbeing endeavors, making it more straightforward for them to spread.

10. Medical Care Foundation and Screening:

• Contrasts in the medical care framework and screening rehearsals among nations can bring about variations in the determination and revealing of parasitic contaminations, influencing the worldwide comprehension of illness dissemination.

Endeavors to control the spread of parasites with regards to globalization include worldwide participation in wellbeing observation, the checking of imported items and vectors, inoculation and treatment programs for explorers and transients, and investigation into sickness elements. The interconnected idea of the world requires a worldwide way to deal with the difficulties presented by the spread of parasitic contamination.

Chapter 7: Indicative and Treatment Difficulties

Developing symptomatic strategies for emerging parasites

The developing symptomatic strategies for arising parasites are urgent for early discovery, observation, and control of the spread of these diseases. Progress in symptomatic methods has worked on the exactness, speed, and availability of parasite location. Here are some developing symptomatic strategies for arising parasites:

1. Sub-atomic Diagnostics:

• Polymerase Chain Response (PCR): PCR methods have changed the diagnosis of parasitic diseases. They offer high awareness and particularity and can identify even low parasite loads.

• Circle-interceded isothermal intensification (light): Light is a fast and touchy sub-atomic strategy for recognizing parasites. It doesn't need particular hardware, making it reasonable for field settings.

• Cutting-edge Sequencing (NGS): NGS innovations consider far-reaching parasite genotyping and the recognizable proof of arising strains and medication obstruction markers.

2. Serological Tests:

• Catalyst Connected Immunosorbent Measures (ELISA): ELISA tests are ordinarily used to recognize antibodies against parasitic antigens. They are especially valuable for diagnosing ongoing contamination.

• Sidelong Stream Measures: Fast demonstrative tests (RDTs) in light of parallel stream innovation are not difficult to use in place-of-care settings and can distinguish explicit antigens or antibodies.

• Multiplex Examines: These tests permit the synchronous recognition of different parasitic diseases, which is beneficial in regions with various co-contaminations.

3. Imaging and Radiology:

• Ultrasound: Ultrasonography is important for diagnosing parasitic contaminations like schistosomiasis and echinococcosis, as it can imagine organ harm brought about by parasites.

• Attractive Reverberation Imaging (X-ray) and Registered Tomography (CT) Outputs: High-level imaging strategies are utilized for diagnosing illnesses like neurocysticercosis.

4. Microscopy:

• Fluorescence Microscopy: Fluorescent colors can improve the perceivability of parasites in clinical examples, making it more straightforward to distinguish them.

• Advanced Microscopy: Computerized magnifying instruments, combined with picture examination programming, empower far-off finding and information sharing for reconnaissance.

5. Antigen Recognition:

• Location of Coursing Antigens: tests that distinguish parasite-explicit antigens in blood or pee, for example, the CATT test for dozing affliction and the purpose-in-care Coursing Cathodic Antigen (CCA) test for schistosomiasis.

6. Biosensors and Nanotechnology:

• The improvement of biosensors and nanotechnology-based tests takes into consideration the fast, delicate, and financially savvy recognition of parasites and their items.

7. Man-made brainpower (computer-based intelligence):

• Computer-based intelligence and AI calculations can break down enormous datasets from symptomatic tests, supporting the identification of emerging patterns and examples in parasite circulation.

8. Telemedicine and Portable Wellbeing (mHealth):

• The utilization of cell phones and telemedicine stages can uphold distant analysis and information sharing, particularly in low-asset and far-off regions.

9. Local Area Wellbeing Laborers (CHWs):

• Preparing and furnishing CHWs with demonstrative devices and methods can further develop admittance to conclusion and treatment in underserved regions.

10. Inventive Example Assortment Strategies:

• Harmless strategies like fingerstick blood tests or pee assortment can make demonstrative methods not so intrusive but rather more satisfactory to patients.

11. Reasons behind Care Testing (POCT):

• POCT gadgets and RDTs empower quick and on-location conclusions, lessening the time between testing and treatment inception.

12. Biosafety and Biosecurity Measures:

• The turn of events and the execution of secure and normalized techniques for taking care of tests, especially in regions with arising and reappearing parasites.

Developing analytic techniques is fundamental for checking and answering arising parasitic contaminations, especially in districts where these diseases are less surely known or less pervasive. These advances assist with guaranteeing that precise and ideal determination is accessible to patients, supporting general wellbeing endeavors to control and forestall the spread of these diseases.

Tending to difficulties in treating drug-safe parasites

Tending to difficulties in treating drug-safe parasites is basic to keeping up with the adequacy of antiparasitic medications and forestalling the spread of safe strains. Drug resistance in parasites can prompt treatment disappointments, expanded dreariness, and general wellbeing concerns. Here are a few procedures for handling drug-safe parasites:

1. Reconnaissance and Checking:

• Standard reconnaissance and observation of parasitic contaminations, drug opposition, and treatment results are fundamental to distinguishing and following the rise of obstruction.

2. Improvement of New Medications:

• Putting resources into innovative work to make new antiparasitic drugs with novel systems of activity can assist with beating opposition.

3. Mix Treatment:

• Utilizing a blend treatment with at least two medications that work through various systems can decrease the risk of oppositional improvement. This approach is known as multidrug treatment (MDT).

4. Portion Improvement:

• Changing medication measurements in view of elements like body weight, age, and hereditary varieties can further develop treatment viability and decrease the risk of obstruction.

5. Treatment Rules:

• Creating and carrying out proof-based treatment rules that consider nearby opposition examples and individual patient attributes is fundamental.

6. Adherence Advancement:

• Elevating patient adherence to treatment regimens is critical. Wellbeing training and support administrations can assist patients with finishing their treatment courses.

7. Elective Conveyance Techniques:

• Investigating elective medication conveyance techniques, like long-acting definitions, can guarantee that patients get the full course of treatment.

8. Vector Control:

• Decreasing the number of inhabitants in sickness vectors, like mosquitoes or snails, can bring down the transmission of parasites and diminish the requirement for therapy.

9. Coordinated Wellbeing Administrations:

• Coordinating antiparasitic treatment with other medical care administrations, for example, inoculation and maternal wellbeing programs, can work on overall wellbeing and prosperity, diminishing the risk of reinfection.

10. Natural Administration:

• Addressing natural factors that contribute to sickness transmission, like water and disinfection enhancements, can supplement drug-based mediations.

11. Examination into Medication Opposition Instruments:

• Examining the atomic and hereditary systems of medication opposition in parasites can give bits of knowledge to creating methodologies to conquer obstruction.

12. Worldwide joint effort:

• Working together with worldwide associations, state-run administrations, and research foundations can facilitate the sharing of information, assets, and mastery in tending to sedate obstruction.

13. Limit Building:

• Preparing medical services Laborers in the analysis and the executives of medication-safe parasites can work on the nature of care and therapy results.

14. Local area commitment:

• Drawing in neighborhood networks into the planning and execution of treatment projects can improve understanding and acknowledgement of mediations.

15. Administrative Measures:

• Carrying out guidelines and oversight of medication quality and appropriation to forestall the sale and utilization of unsatisfactory or fake antiparasitic drugs.

16. Schooling and Mindfulness:

• bringing issues to light among medical care experts and general society about the significance of fitting medication use, the dangers of obstruction, and the requirement for reasonable endorsing.

Tending to sedate safe parasites requires a multi-layered approach that encompasses drug improvement, treatment systems, reconnaissance, and local area contribution. By carrying out these methodologies, the general wellbeing of the local area can attempt to forestall and oversee drug opposition in parasitic contaminations and keep up with the adequacy of accessible medicines.

Chapter 8: Observation and Counteraction

The significance of observation in following arising dangers

Observation is of central significance in following arising dangers, including arising parasitic contaminations. It assumes a vital role in early discovery, observation, and reaction to these dangers. Here's the reason why reconnaissance is fundamental:

1. Early Discovery: Reconnaissance takes into consideration the early location of arising dangers. By ceaselessly checking patterns in illnesses and medical issues, general wellbeing specialists can recognize strange examples and speedily research likely episodes.

2. Quick Reaction: Early discovery empowers a quick and facilitated reaction to arising dangers. General wellbeing organizations can start control measures, execute treatment conventions, and convey assets to contain the danger before it heightens.

3. Forestall Spread: Reconnaissance helps in distinguishing the source and method of transmission of arising diseases. This data is crucial for executing designated intercessions to forestall additional spread.

4. Checking Patterns: Reconnaissance gives a verifiable viewpoint on the movement of arising dangers. Understanding how these dangers develop after some time helps in asset allocation and distribution.

5. Risk Appraisal: Observation information empowers general wellbeing authorities to evaluate the risk to the populace and arrive at informed conclusions about the requirement for

mediations, for example, inoculation missions or vector control measures.

6. Asset Distribution: Reconnaissance information guides the assignment of assets, including staff, subsidizing, and clinical supplies, to regions most impacted by arising dangers.

7. Innovative work: Information gathered through observation projects can illuminate research endeavors to grasp the science, transmission, and conduct of arising parasites, helping with the advancement of demonstrative instruments, medicines, and avoidance methodologies.

8. General Wellbeing Approaches: Observation educates the advancement regarding general wellbeing arrangements and rules to address arising dangers. This incorporates suggestions for medical care suppliers, tourism warnings, and immunization programs.

9. Worldwide Joint effort: observation information is imparted to worldwide wellbeing associations and adjoining nations to work with cooperative reactions to arising dangers that might have cross-line suggestions.

10. Public Mindfulness: Reconnaissance information can be utilized to teach people in general about the dangers of arising dangers, empowering people to avoid potential risks and look for ideal clinical consideration.

11. Limit Building: Observation programs add to the advancement of nearby medical services foundations and fortify the limit of medical services laborers ability to distinguish and answer arising dangers.

12. Information for Exploration: Reconnaissance information acts as an important asset for epidemiological and general wellbeing research, assisting scientists with better grasping the elements of arising diseases.

13. Responsibility and Straightforwardness: Powerful reconnaissance programs advance responsibility and straightforwardness in the medical services framework, permitting people in general to screen their reactions to arising dangers.

14. Readiness for Future Dangers: Reconnaissance gives experiences into the variables that contribute to the rise of dangers, empowering readiness for future occasions.

With regards to arising parasitic contaminations, reconnaissance is crucial for tending to sicknesses like jungle fever, dengue fever, dismissed tropical infections, and recently recognized parasites. By following these dangers, general wellbeing frameworks can more readily safeguard the wellbeing and prosperity of networks, forestall plagues, and answer arising difficulties in a convenient and successful way.

Protection measures and control systems

Protection measures and control systems for arising parasitic contaminations are fundamental to alleviating the effect of these illnesses on general wellbeing. These actions mean to diminish transmission, safeguard weak populations, and, at last, forestall the spread of parasitic diseases. Here are a few vital methodologies for forestalling and controlling arising parasitic diseases:

1. Vector Control:

• Executing vector control measures to lessen the number of inhabitants with illness conveying vectors (e.g., mosquitoes, sandflies, snails).

• Utilization of insect-poison-treated bed nets and indoor lingering splashing for intestinal sickness and other vector-borne infections.

2. Further developed sanitation and cleanliness:

• Guaranteeing admittance to safe drinking water, appropriate disinfection offices, and cleanliness instruction to lessen waterborne and waste oral parasitic diseases.

3. Mass Medication Organization (MDA):

• Carrying out MDA projects to manage preventive prescriptions for populations in danger in endemic regions. This methodology is utilized for illnesses like lymphatic filariasis and schistosomiasis.

4. Vaccination:

• Creating and advancing antibodies for parasitic diseases. The improvement of a jungle fever immunization, for instance, addresses a critical headway in illness counteraction.

5. Wellbeing, Schooling, and Conduct Change:

• bringing issues to light about parasitic contamination, their transmission, and preventive measures.

• Advancing conduct change, like the utilization of defensive attire and the evasion of high-risk regions.

6. Further developed Conclusion and Reconnaissance:

• Extending admittance to exact demonstrative instruments for early identification.

• Reinforcing reconnaissance frameworks to screen illness drifts and distinguish arising dangers.

7. Preventive Chemotherapy:

• Regulating antiparasitic medications for populations in danger as a preventive measure.

• Designated treatment of school-matured kids, pregnant ladies, and other high-risk gatherings.

8. Local area commitment:

• including neighborhood networks in the planning and execution of control programs.

• Utilizing people group wellbeing laborers to convey training and treatment administrations.

9. Innovative work:

• Supporting investigation into new indicative apparatuses, medicines, and control methodologies.

• researching drug obstruction and arising parasites to direct mediations.

10. Worldwide joint effort:

• Teaming up with worldwide wellbeing associations, adjoining nations, and accomplices to organize endeavors and offer prescribed procedures.

11. Coordinated Wellbeing Administrations:

• Incorporating the avoidance and control of parasitic diseases with other medical care administrations, for example, maternal and child wellbeing programs.

12. Scourge Readiness and Reaction:

• Creating emergency courses of action and reaction instruments for tending to flare-ups of arising parasitic contaminations.

13. Environmental Change Transformation:

• Planning for the effect of environmental change on the dispersion of parasites and their vectors.

14. Promotion and Financing:

• Upholding expanded subsidizing and assets to help parasitic contamination avoidance and control endeavors.

15. Treatment of Comorbidities:

• Tending to comorbid conditions, for example, HIV or a lack of healthy sustenance, that can worsen the effects of parasitic diseases.

Protection measures and control procedures ought to be customized to the particular qualities of the arising parasitic contamination and the nearby setting. A complete and multidisciplinary approach, including legislatures, medical care suppliers, scientists, and impacted networks, is fundamental for powerful counteraction and control. These procedures aim not exclusively to decrease the weight of parasitic diseases but additionally to work on the general wellbeing and prosperity of impacted populations.

Chapter 9: The Job of Exploration and Development

Exploration and advancement assume an essential part in the area of parasitology. By propelling comprehension, we might interpret parasitic diseases, develop new devices and systems for determination, treatment, and counteraction, and tend to arising difficulties. Here are a few vital parts of the job of exploration and development in parasitology:

1. Grasping Parasitic Science:

• Research assists researchers with disentangling the science, life cycles, and instruments of parasites, giving experiences into their way of behaving and collaborations with them.

2. Drug Improvement and Medication Obstruction:

• Research drives the advancement of new antiparasitic drugs and the investigation of medication targets. It is fundamental for understanding and fighting medication obstruction in parasites.

3. Vaccines:

• Creative exploration endeavors are basic for the advancement of immunizations against parasitic diseases like intestinal sickness and schistosomiasis.

4. Indicative Apparatuses:

• Research prompts the development of more precise, fast, and savvy demonstrative strategies for parasitic diseases, upgrading early identification.

5. Vector Control:

• Advancements in vector control techniques, like the improvement of novel insect sprays or hereditary changes in sickness vectors, contribute to lessening illness transmission.

6. The study of disease transmission and illness display:

• Research helps in planning the dissemination of parasitic diseases and displaying their spread, supporting designated mediations and asset allotment.

7. Genomic and Atomic Examinations:

• Progresses in genomics and sub-atomic science empower researchers to concentrate on the hereditary qualities of parasites, which can illuminate drug improvement and opposition systems.

8. Coordinated Approaches:

• Research upholds the improvement of incorporated techniques that join numerous intercessions, for example, drug treatment, vector control, and wellbeing schooling.

9. Environmental Change Transformation:

• Understanding the effect of environmental change on the appropriation of parasites and their vectors is urgent for creating versatile procedures.

10. One Wellbeing Approach:

• Research advances the One Wellbeing approach, which perceives the interconnectedness of human, creature, and natural wellbeing with regards to parasitic diseases.

11. Social and Conduct Exploration:

• Researching the social and conduct factors that impact parasitic contamination transmission and control measures can illuminate general wellbeing efforts and conduct change mediations.

12. Schooling and Limit Building:

• Research adds to the preparation and limits the work of researchers, medical service workers, and networks engaged in parasitology.

13. Worldwide coordinated effort:

• Cooperative examination drives, including numerous nations and associations, work with the sharing of information, assets, and mastery to handle parasitic contaminations on a worldwide scale.

14. Development in Treatment Conveyance:

• Development in medical services conveyance techniques, for example, telemedicine and versatile wellbeing (mHealth) advancements, can improve admission to therapy and follow-up care.

15. Public Mindfulness:

• Research discoveries can be utilized to raise public awareness about the dangers of parasitic diseases and the significance of preventive measures.

16. Promotion and Financing:

• Research gives the proof base to support endeavors pointed toward getting financing and assets for parasitology exploration and mediation.

In summary, examination and advancement are fundamental for propelling our insight into parasitic contaminations, creating successful apparatuses and systems for control and avoidance, and tending to arising difficulties in parasitology. These endeavors are instrumental in lessening the worldwide weight of parasitic illnesses and working on the wellbeing and prosperity of impacted populations.

Developments and leaps forward in combating arising dangers

In the battle against arising dangers, including parasitic contamination, developments and leap forwards played a significant role in working on our capacity to identify, forestall, and control these illnesses. Here are a few striking developments and leaps forward:

1. Genomic Sequencing:

• The headway of genomic sequencing advances has empowered the fast identification and portrayal of arising parasites. This has been significant for figuring out their science and creating designated mediations.

2. Intestinal sickness immunity (RTS):

• The turn of events and endorsement of the RTS,S jungle fever immunization address a critical leap forward in the counteraction of one of the world's deadliest parasitic sicknesses.

3. CRISPR-Based Quality Altering:

• CRISPR innovation is being investigated for the hereditary change of illness vectors, like mosquitoes, to lessen their capacity to communicate parasites like intestinal sickness.

4. Mark-of-Care Diagnostics:

• Advancements in reason-behind-care analytic tests, including fast demonstrative tests (RDTs) and sub-atomic examinations, have worked on the early discovery of parasitic diseases in asset-restricted settings.

5. Drug Revelation:

• Propels in drug revelation advances and the improvement of novel mixtures have prompted the formation of more compelling antiparasitic drugs.

6. Computer-based intelligence and AI:

• AI calculations are being utilized to break down enormous datasets and anticipate infection episodes, as well as to foster symptomatic devices and advance treatment regimens.

7. Bug spray-treated bed nets:

• The boundless conveyance of insect spray-treated bed nets has essentially diminished the transmission of intestinal sickness and other vector-borne illnesses.

8. Natural Control of Vectors:

• Creative organic control techniques, for example, the utilization of Wolbachia microorganisms to decrease mosquito populations, show a guarantee of diminishing illness transmission.

9. Environment Demonstrating:

• Refined environment models permit analysts to anticipate the effect of environmental change on the dissemination of parasites and their vectors, helping with readiness.

10. Local Area Wellbeing Laborers (CHWs):

• Utilizing CHWs outfitted with cell phones for information assortment and treatment organization has further developed admittance to medical services in far-off regions.

11. Telemedicine and mHealth:

• The utilization of telemedicine and versatile wellbeing advancements has extended access to medical care benefits and further developed sickness reconnaissance in remote and underserved locales.

12. Social and Conduct Intercessions:

• Conducting science research has prompted the improvement of viable general wellbeing efforts and the conduct of change interventions to advance preventive measures.

13. Public-Private Associations:

• Cooperative endeavors between state-run administrations, non-legislative associations, and drug organizations have sped up the turn of events and the dispersion of antibodies and medicines.

14. Coordinated Approaches:

• Imaginative systems that coordinate medical care administrations, vector control, and local area commitment have worked on the adequacy of parasitic disease control.

15. Worldwide Wellbeing Security:

• The advancement of worldwide wellbeing security structures and the execution of Global Wellbeing Guidelines upgrade worldwide participation in identifying and answering arising dangers.

These developments and leaps forward embody the headway made in combating arising parasitic contaminations and other wellbeing dangers. They highlight the significance of examination, innovation, and cooperative endeavors in the worldwide battle against these illnesses. Nonetheless, continuous exploration and advancement are urgent to address new difficulties and arising dangers in parasitology.

Conclusion

The area of parasitology encompasses the investigation of parasitic creatures, their effect on human and creature wellbeing, and the improvement of systems to forestall, analyze, and treat parasitic diseases. Here are key discoveries connected with parasitology:

1. Definition and Significance of Parasitic Diseases:

• Parasitic contaminations are brought about by different living beings, including protozoa, helminths, and arthropods. They are a huge worldwide wellbeing concern, especially in low-asset districts, and can bring about a large number of illnesses.

2. Arising Dangers in Parasitic Diseases:

• Arising dangers in parasitic contaminations incorporate the presence of new parasitic species, the spread of medication opposition, changes in vector conveyance, and the impact of variables like environmental change and urbanization.

3. Job of Globalization in Parasitic Diseases:

• Globalization, portrayed by expanded worldwide travel, exchange, and interconnectedness, has worked with the spread of parasites and the sicknesses they cause. Worldwide travel, relocation, and the development of products and vectors can contribute to the spread of parasitic diseases.

4. Analysis and Treatment Difficulties:

• Diagnosing parasitic contamination can be difficult because of elements like asymptomatic transporters, restricted admittance to analytic devices, and clinical side effects. Treatment challenges incorporate medication opposition, restricted treatment choices, and comorbid conditions.

5. Advancing Analytic Strategies:

• Propels in analytic strategies, like atomic diagnostics, serological tests, and imaging procedures, have worked on the exactness and availability of parasite discovery.

6. Tending to Difficulties in Treating Medication-Safe Parasites:

• Tending to sedate safe parasites requires reconnaissance, the advancement of new medications, mix treatment, portion enhancement, and designated treatment programs. A multisectoral joint effort is fundamental.

7. Significance of Reconnaissance in Following Arising Dangers:

• Observation is imperative for early identification, fast reaction, and the checking of arising parasitic diseases. It gives basic information to gamble with appraisal, asset assignment, and global coordinated effort.

8. Deterrent Measures and Control Systems:

• Safeguard measures and control procedures include vector control, further developed sterilization and cleanliness, mass medication organization, immunization, wellbeing schooling, further developed findings, and innovative work. These systems mean to diminish transmission and safeguard weak populations.

9. Job of Exploration and Development in Parasitology:

• Exploration and advancement are major for grasping parasitic contaminations, growing new medications, diagnostics, and immunizations, and tending to arising difficulties. Genomic sequencing, simulated intelligence, and place-of-care diagnostics are among the creative devices changing the field.

10. Advancements and Forward Sights in Combating Arising Dangers:

• Advancements and leaps forward in parasitology incorporate the improvement of jungle fever immunization, CRISPR-based quality altering for vector control, place-of-care diagnostics, and high-level medication revelation strategies. These advancements are changing the fate of parasitic disease control.

These key discoveries feature the diverse idea of parasitology and the basic job it plays in worldwide wellbeing. Continuous examination, development, and cooperative endeavors are fundamental for handling arising parasitic diseases and further developing the prosperity of impacted populations.

The significance of worldwide participation in overseeing parasitic contaminations

Worldwide participation is of principal significance in overseeing parasitic contaminations for a few convincing reasons:

1. Forestalling Cross-Boundary Transmission: Parasitic diseases don't perceive political lines. Collaboration between nations is significant to forestall the cross-line transmission of parasites and contain arising dangers successfully.

2. Early Location and Reaction: Convenient identification of arising diseases frequently requires worldwide information sharing and cooperation. Early reaction measures can assist with keeping restricted episodes from becoming pandemics.

3. Asset Distribution: Worldwide collaboration works with a fair allotment of assets to battle parasitic diseases. Asset-rich nations can uphold asset-unlucky districts, but they are abandoned to guarantee that no populace.

4. Data Sharing and Reconnaissance: Sharing data on illness patterns, arising dangers, and medication opposition is indispensable for informed independent direction and facilitated reactions.

5. Antibody and Medication Improvement: Cooperative exploration endeavors, frequently including numerous nations, speed up the advancement of antibodies, antiparasitic drugs, and demonstrative apparatuses. This prompts more viable and available mediations.

6. Limit Building: Coordinated effort advances the trading of information and aptitude between nations. It upholds limits on working in research, diagnostics, treatment, and medical services conveyance.

7. Helpful Help: Worldwide participation considers the arrangement of helpful help with locales impacted by emerging parasitic diseases. This incorporates clinical supplies, treatment, and support for impacted populations.

8. Global Wellbeing Guidelines (IHR): Consistence with IHR cultivates worldwide participation by setting principles for infection observation, detailing, and reaction. It fortifies the worldwide wellbeing security structure.

9. Research Cooperation: Cooperative examination drives, including researchers from different nations, improve the comprehension of parasitic contamination, drug opposition, and arising dangers.

10. Preventive Measures: Carrying out preventive measures like immunization missions and vector control is much more viable when led on a territorial or worldwide scale.

11. Reconnaissance and Checking: Improved observation frameworks that track the development of arising dangers require global coordination. This is especially significant in areas where observation foundations are restricted.

12. Multilateral Associations: Worldwide associations, like the World Wellbeing Association (WHO), work with worldwide collaboration by organizing endeavors, giving specialized direction, and pushing for subsidizing.

13. Political Responsibility: Undeniable levels of political responsibility and collaboration are important to resolve cross-cutting issues like environmental change, urbanization, and populace developments that influence the spread of parasitic diseases.

14. Information Sharing for Exploration and Control: Open access to explore information and discoveries advances logical cooperation and the improvement of creative arrangements.

15. Worldwide Wellbeing Value: Participation in overseeing arising parasitic diseases is a sign of worldwide wellbeing value. It guarantees that all countries approach the assets and backing expected to safeguard the wellbeing of their populations.

16. Emergency Reaction: In case of significant flare-ups or scourges, global participation can offer prompt help and assets to impacted nations.

In summary, worldwide collaboration is fundamental in overseeing arising parasitic diseases. It empowers countries to share their assets and information and endeavors to completely handle these difficulties. By cooperating, nations can further develop readiness, improve infectious prevention, and defend the wellbeing and prosperity of individuals around the world.

www.ingramcontent.com/pod-product-compliance
Lightning Source LLC
Chambersburg PA
CBHW062254290526
45794CB00006B/2539